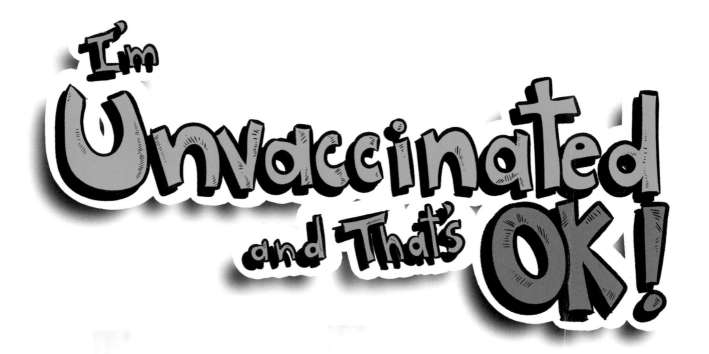

Written by Dr. Shannon Kroner
Illustrated by Manfred Calderón

To the parents who personally know vaccine injury; I hear you.
To the children who have suffered vaccine injury; I see you.
To the vaccinated, partially vaccinated, and unvaccinated; the choice should always remain your own.

This book is dedicated to my mom for always being in my corner
and showing me what it means to be a mama bear. -S.K.

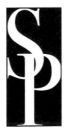

Skyhorse Publishing

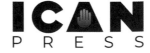

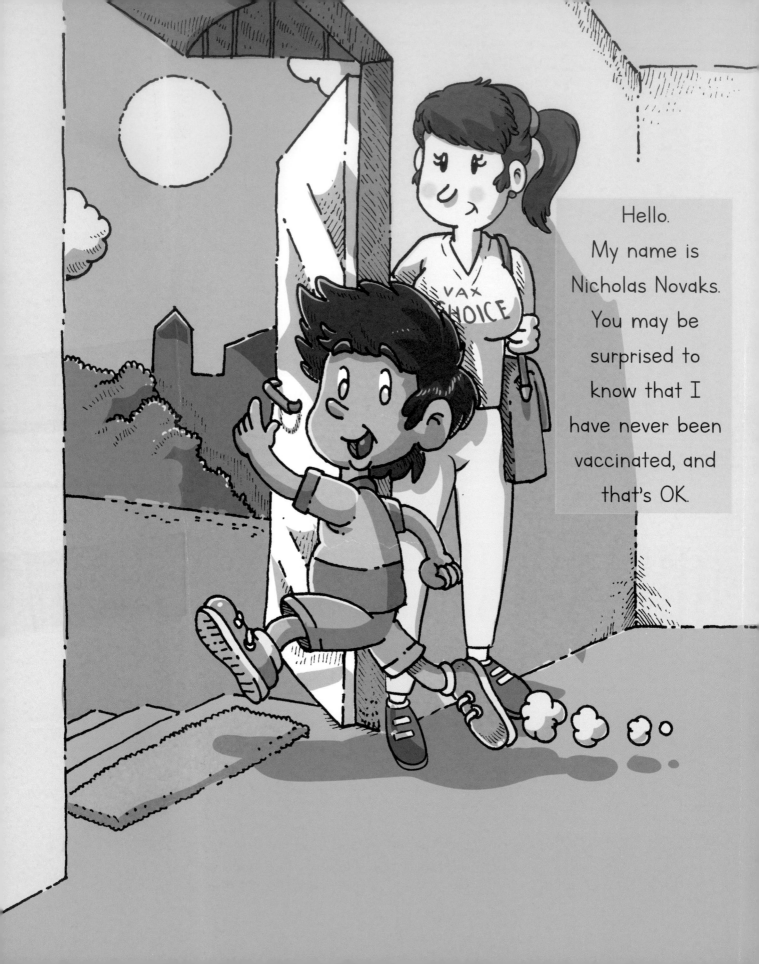

Hello. My name is Nicholas Novaks. You may be surprised to know that I have never been vaccinated, and that's OK.

Some of my friends get vaccinated when they go to the doctor because that is the decision their parents make for them.

My mom and dad say that we have the freedom to choose what goes into our bodies.

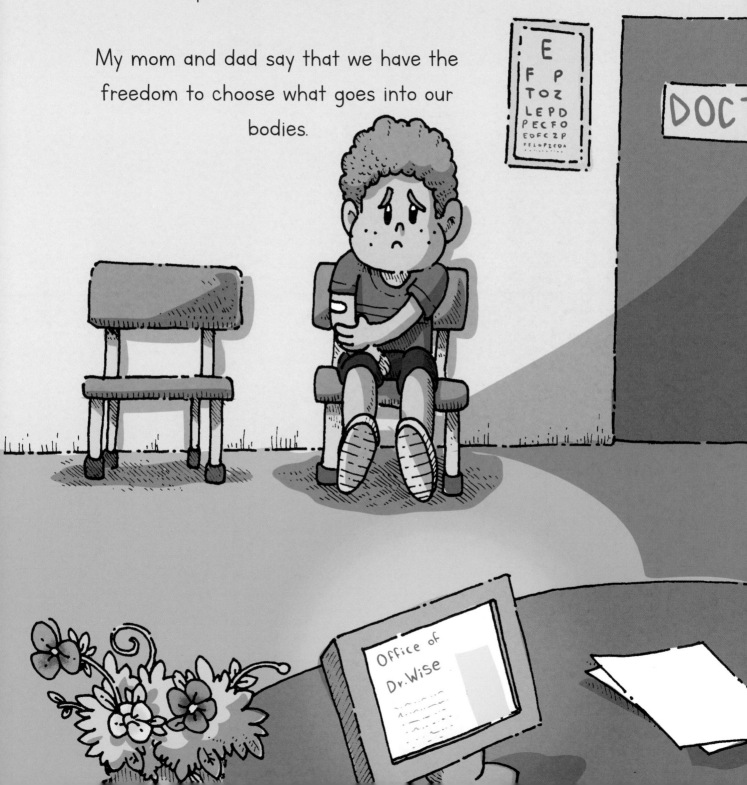

When my sister was a baby my parents followed the recommended childhood vaccine schedule. Unfortunately, after a round of shots she had a very bad reaction.

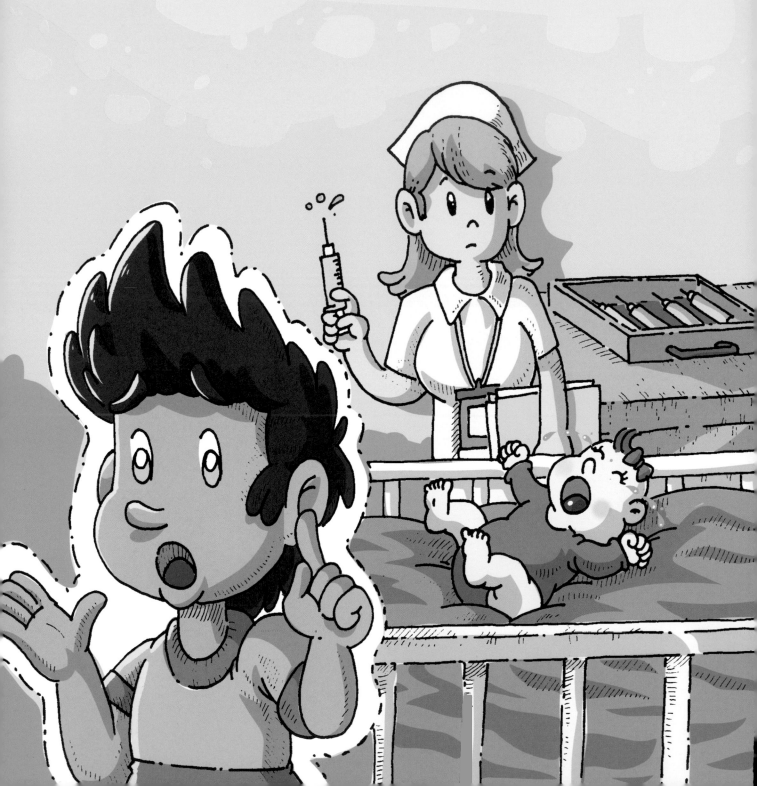

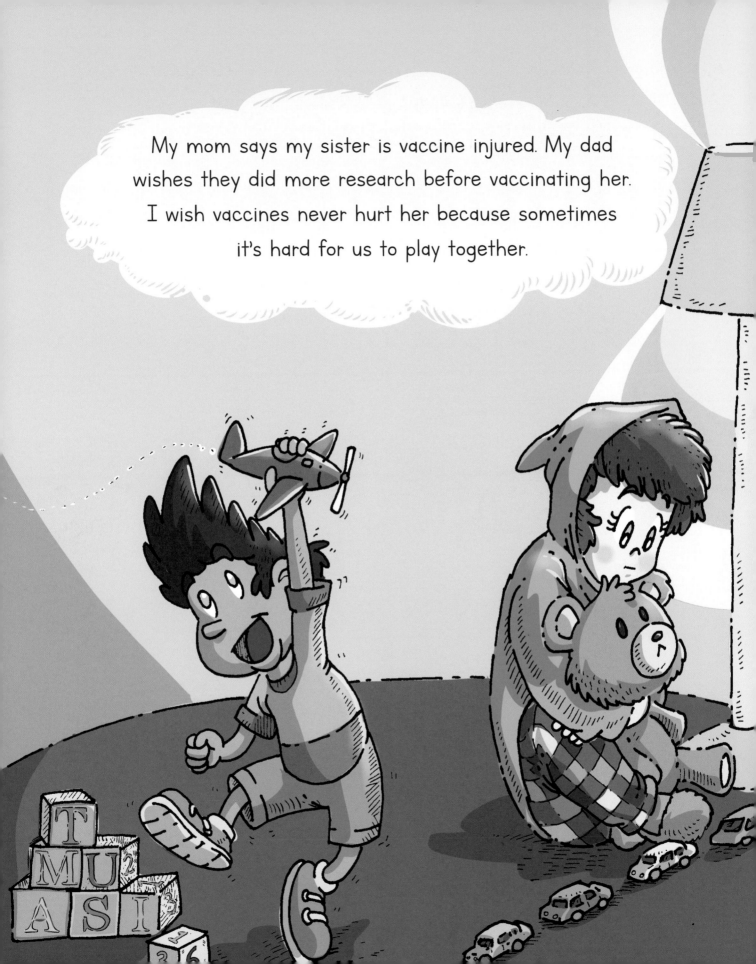

People often ask why my sister doesn't speak or make eye contact.

It's because she has something called autism.

Many doctors say that vaccines don't cause autism; but that's not necessarily true. Vaccines have been known to cause neurological issues and damage to the brain, which can lead to delays in development and other complications.

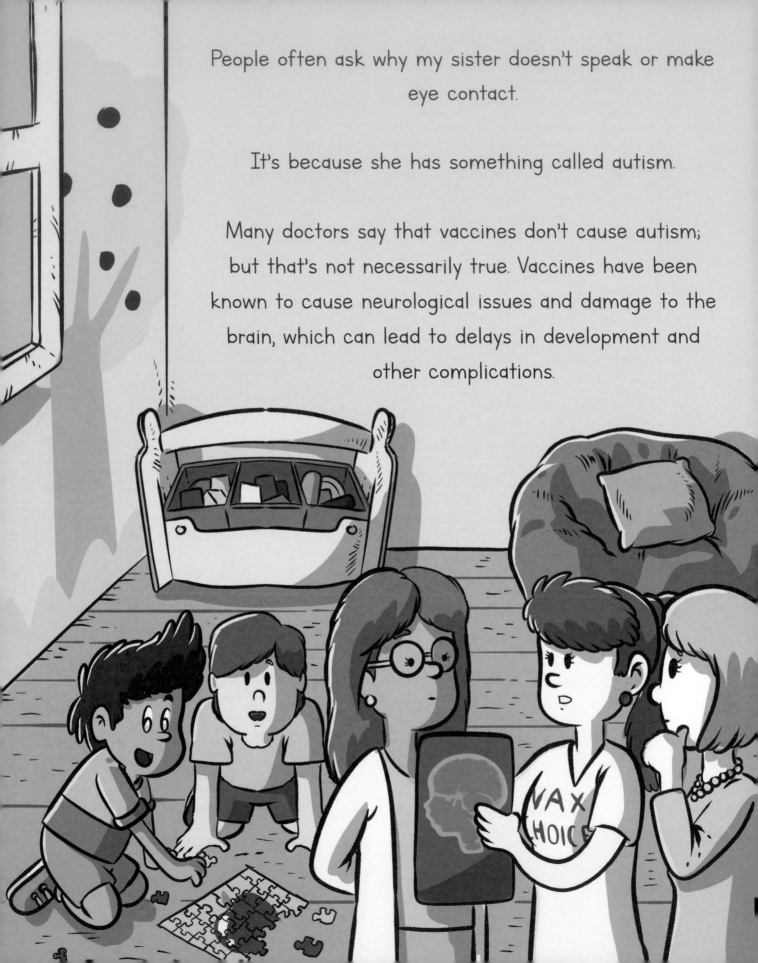

My parents have explained that vaccines caused my sister to have a high fever and brain swelling. Brain swelling is called encephalitis and is a potential adverse reaction that may occur with vaccination. Almost 70% of kids with autism have experienced brain swelling.

These vaccine reactions caused changes in my sister's behavior which led to her autism diagnosis.

This is one of many reasons why my parents won't vaccinate me and have stopped vaccinating my sister.

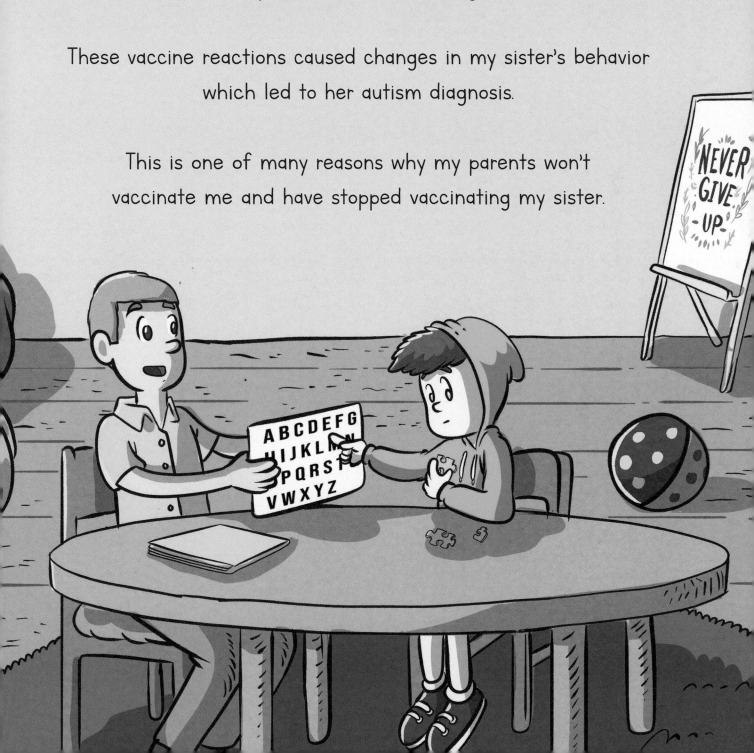

Some people worry that I will get them sick because I'm not vaccinated, but I can't spread a sickness that I don't have. Besides, if they've been vaccinated and their vaccines work, then they shouldn't feel the need to avoid me.

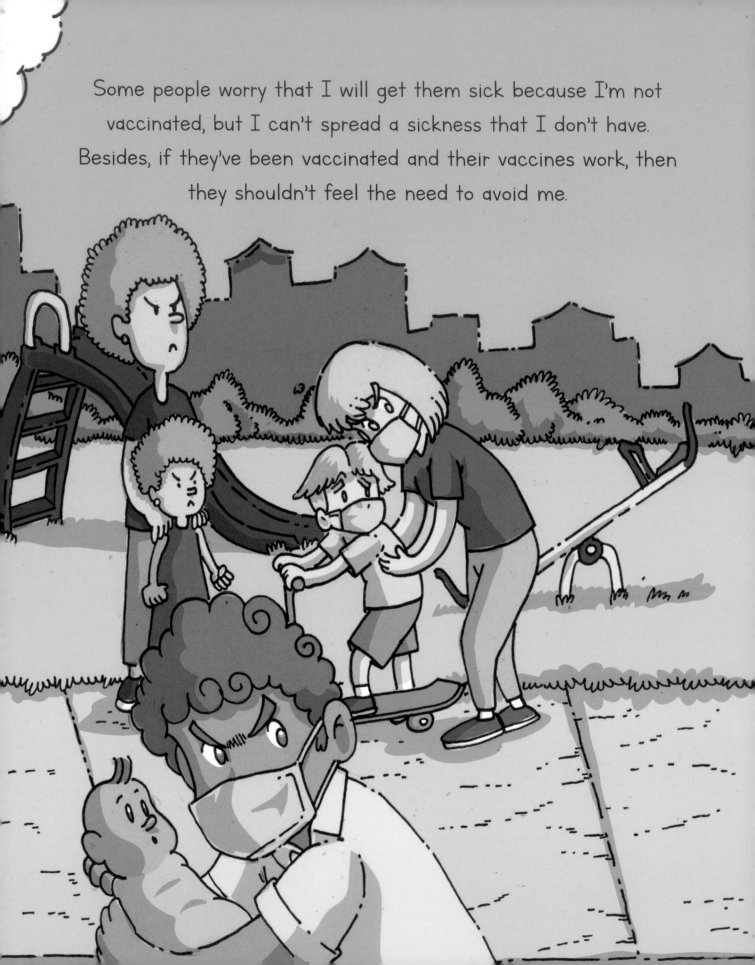

Fortunately, I rarely get sick. My parents say it's because I have a healthy immune system. But if I do get a sniffle or a cough, they make sure I am better before allowing me to play with my friends.

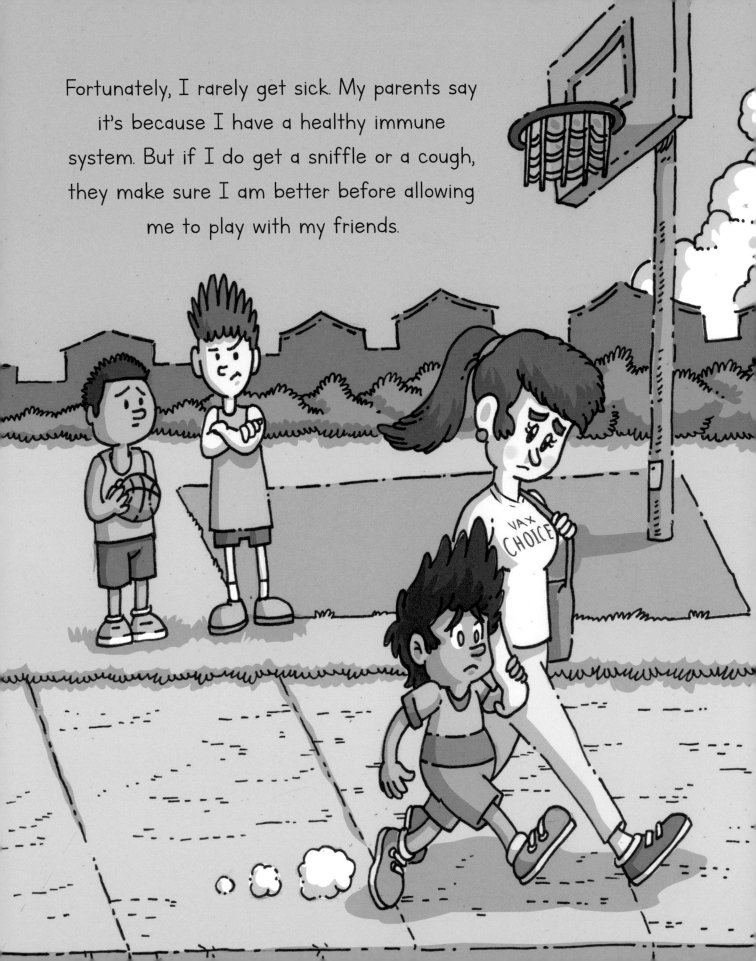

Keeping me and my sister healthy is very important to my parents.

Since a huge part of our immune system exists in our digestive tract, they make sure most of the food we eat is organic.

Organic means that the food isn't grown with toxic fertilizers or sprayed with harmful chemicals.

We also take vitamins, drink plenty of water, get lots of fresh air, and exercise to stay healthy.

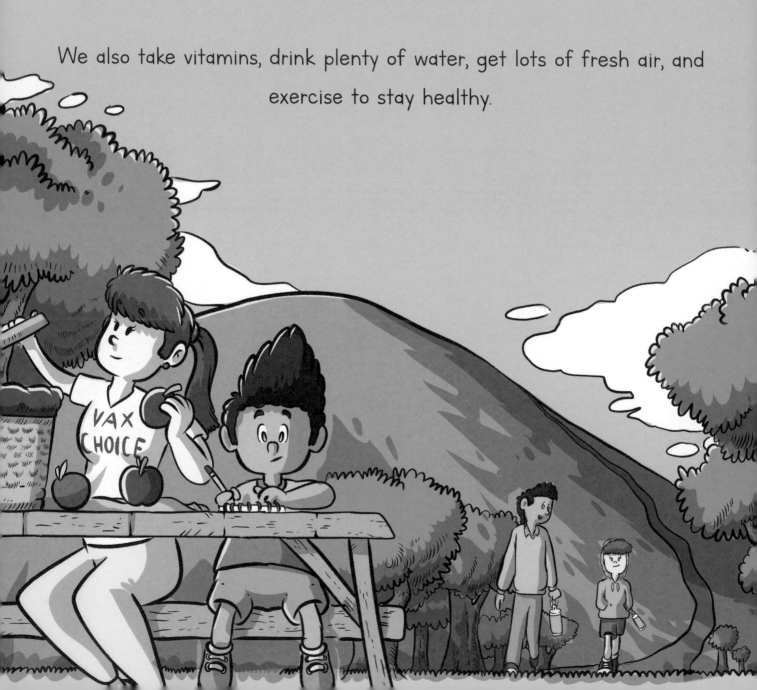

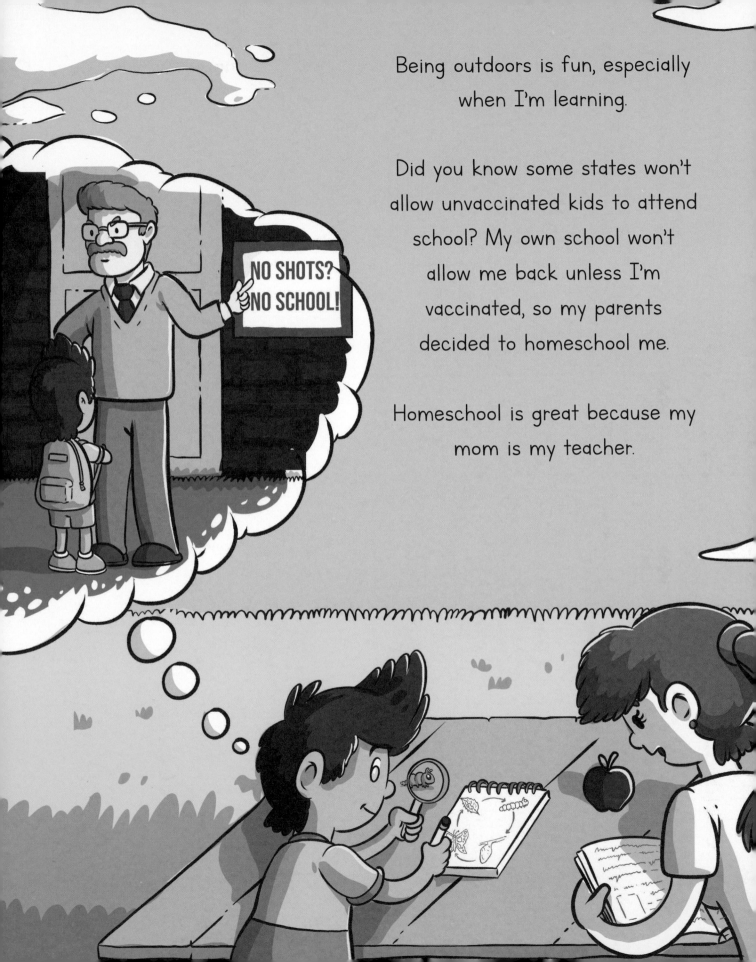

Being outdoors is fun, especially when I'm learning.

Did you know some states won't allow unvaccinated kids to attend school? My own school won't allow me back unless I'm vaccinated, so my parents decided to homeschool me.

Homeschool is great because my mom is my teacher.

NO SHOTS? NO SCHOOL!

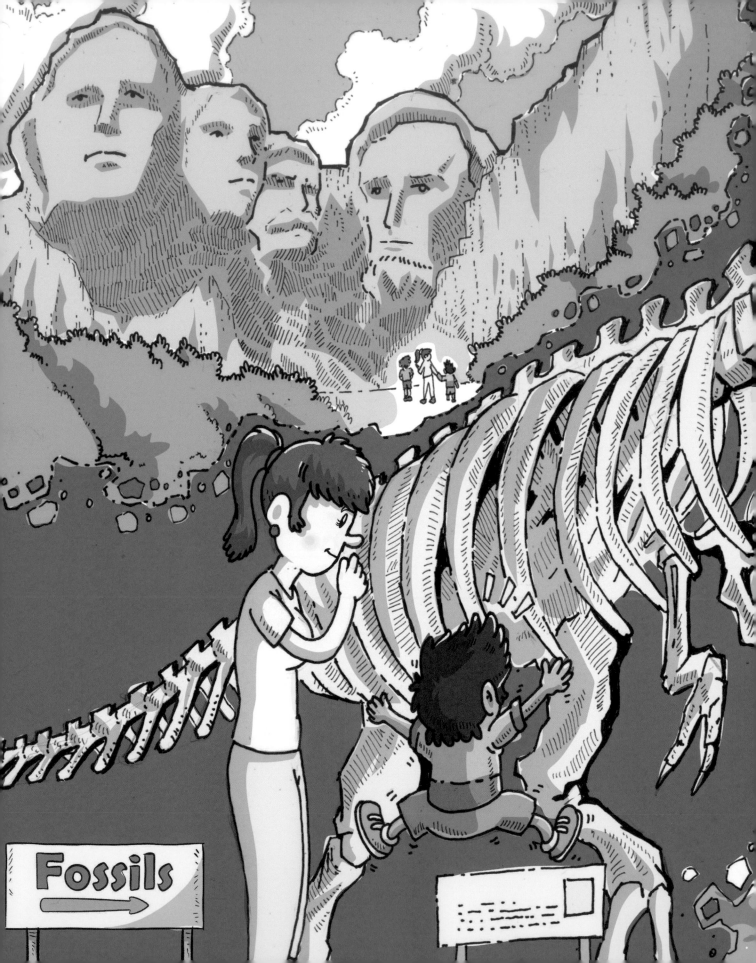

Fossils →

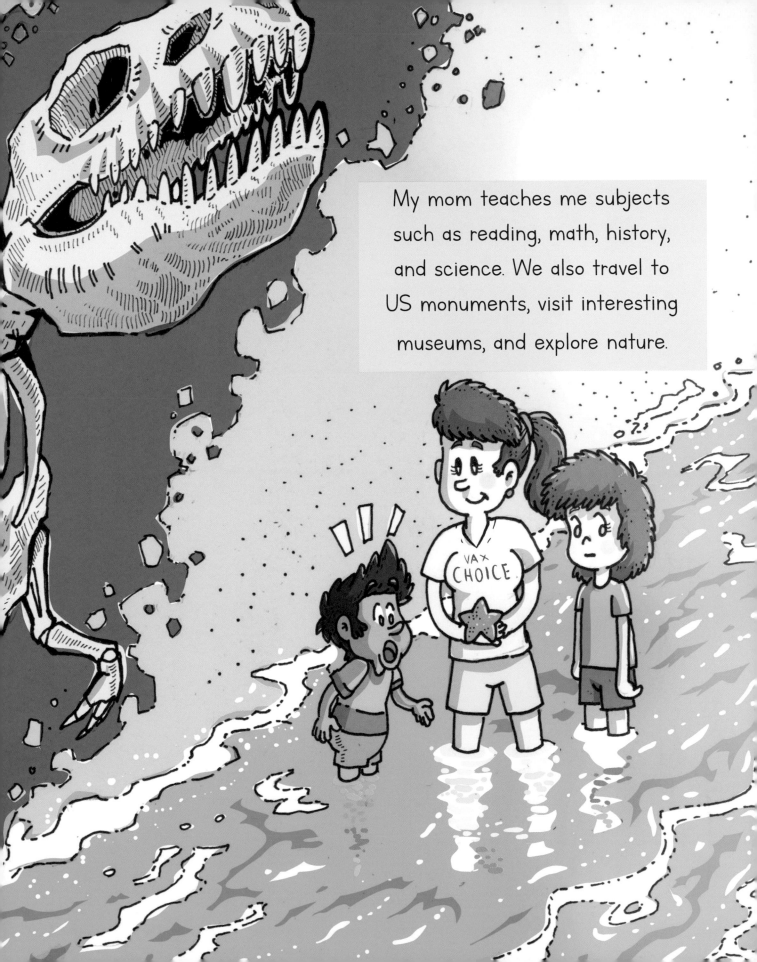

My mom teaches me subjects such as reading, math, history, and science. We also travel to US monuments, visit interesting museums, and explore nature.

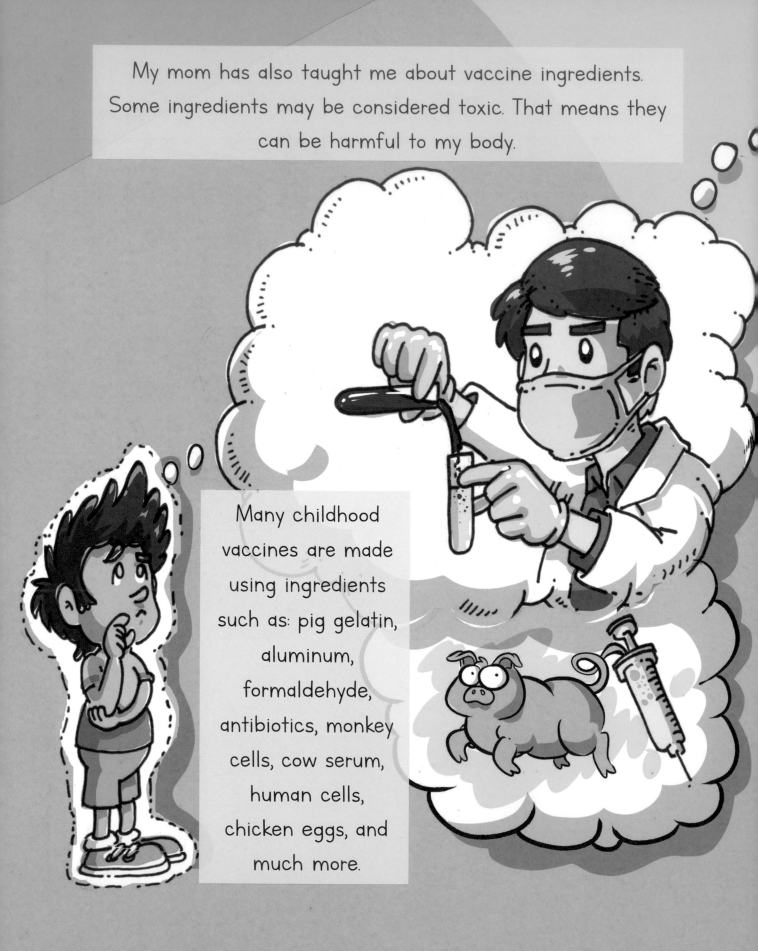

My mom has also taught me about vaccine ingredients. Some ingredients may be considered toxic. That means they can be harmful to my body.

Many childhood vaccines are made using ingredients such as: pig gelatin, aluminum, formaldehyde, antibiotics, monkey cells, cow serum, human cells, chicken eggs, and much more.

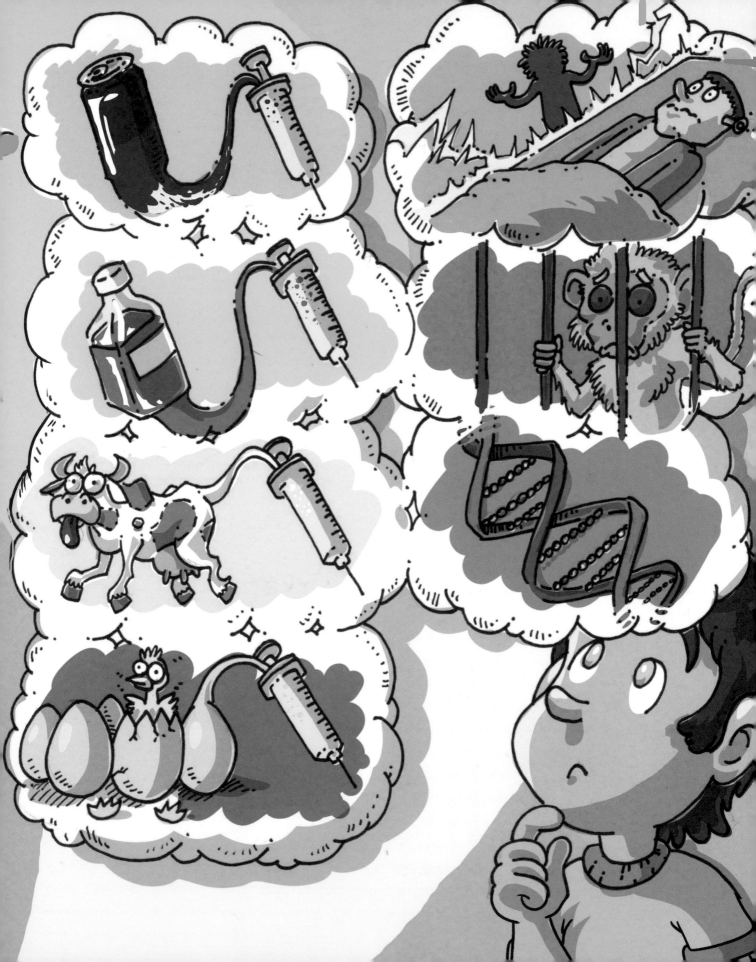

Some people may think it's risky not getting vaccinated, but my parents have learned a lot, weighed the risks, and aren't making these decisions alone. After my sister's vaccine injury, they met with many doctors in search of one who listened to their concerns, understood our family values, and honored freedom of choice.

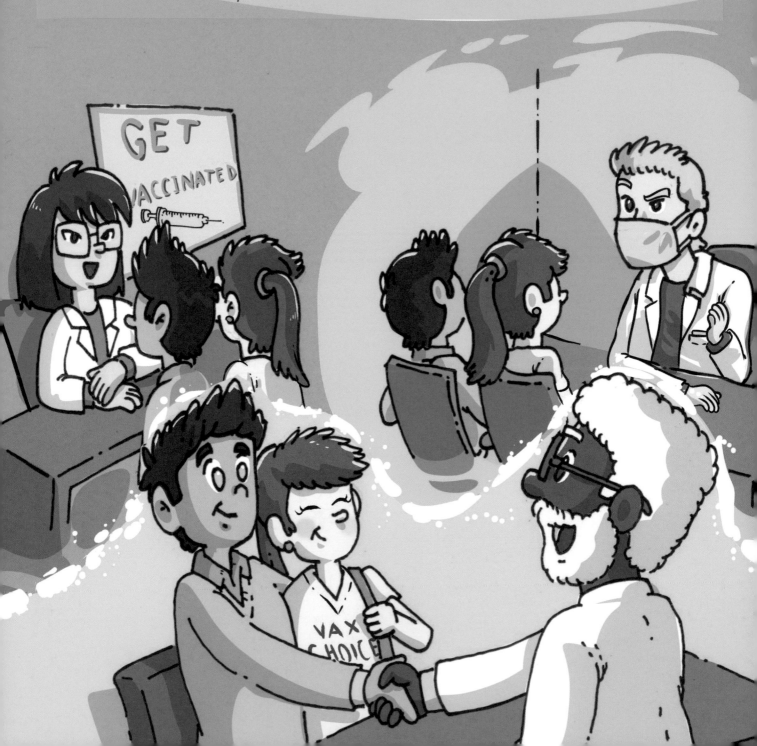

Finding a doctor who is the right fit for our family has been very important because my parents need to feel comfortable speaking about vaccines with someone they trust.
We knew we found the right doctor when he also shared concerns about the rapidly growing vaccine schedule.

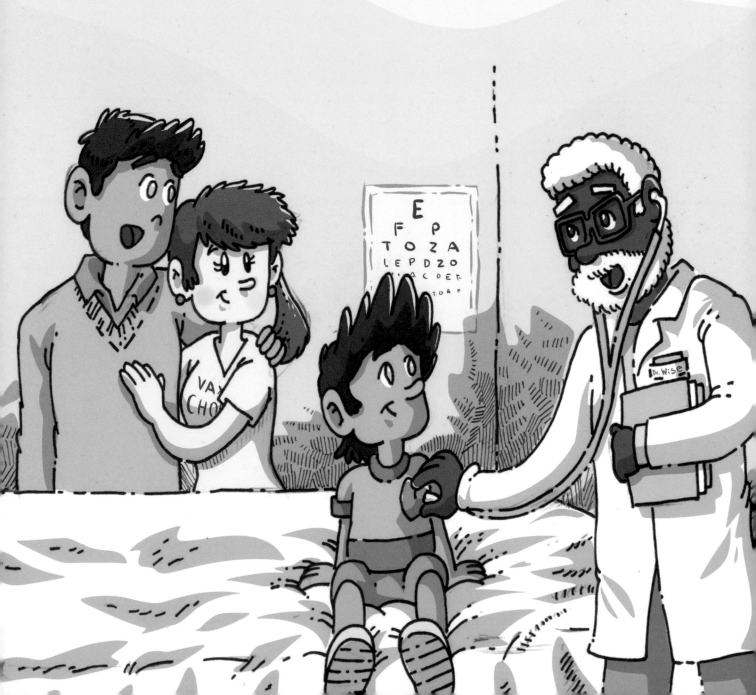

The childhood vaccine schedule has grown a lot over the years. Doctors, scientists, and public health researchers continue adding new vaccines to the schedule without ever testing them in combination to see how all these vaccines interact with each other. Would you believe, I'm expected to get almost one hundred doses of seventeen vaccines by my eighteenth birthday?!

That's a lot!

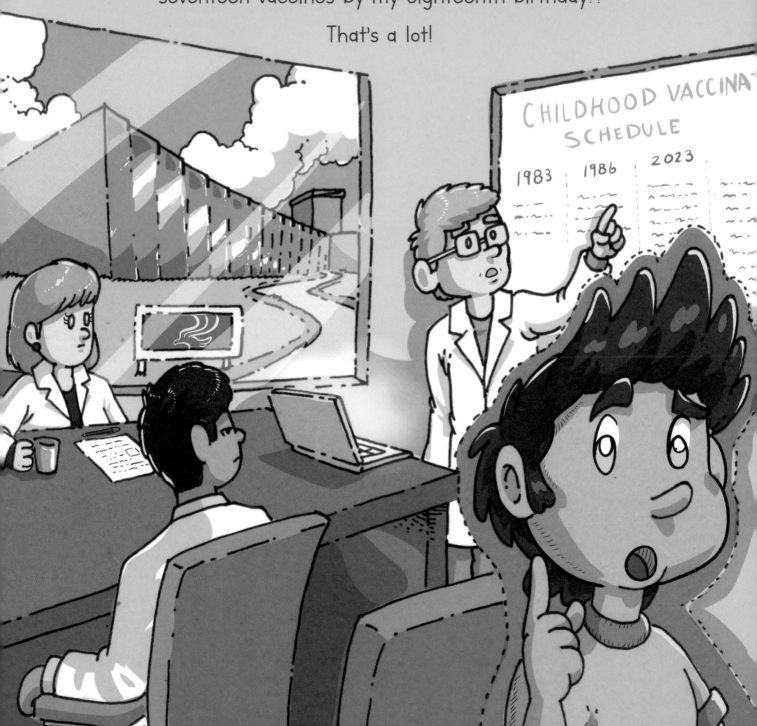

My parents are especially concerned that vaccines have no liability. This means if a vaccine injures me, my sister, or anyone else, no one can be held responsible; not even the companies who made them or the doctors and nurses who give them.

I don't think that's fair because my parents have always taught me to take responsibility for my actions.

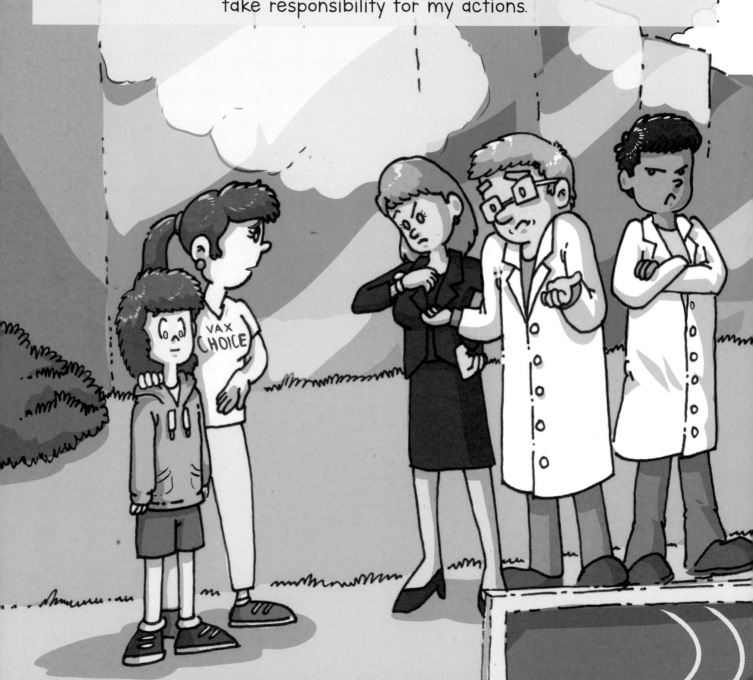

I've also wondered why everyone is expected to get the same vaccines even though we are all different.

Some of my friends are taller than me. Some of my friends are smaller than me. We are different shapes and sizes. We each have our own family medical history and are all genetically different.

So, why are our diversities never considered when it comes to vaccines?

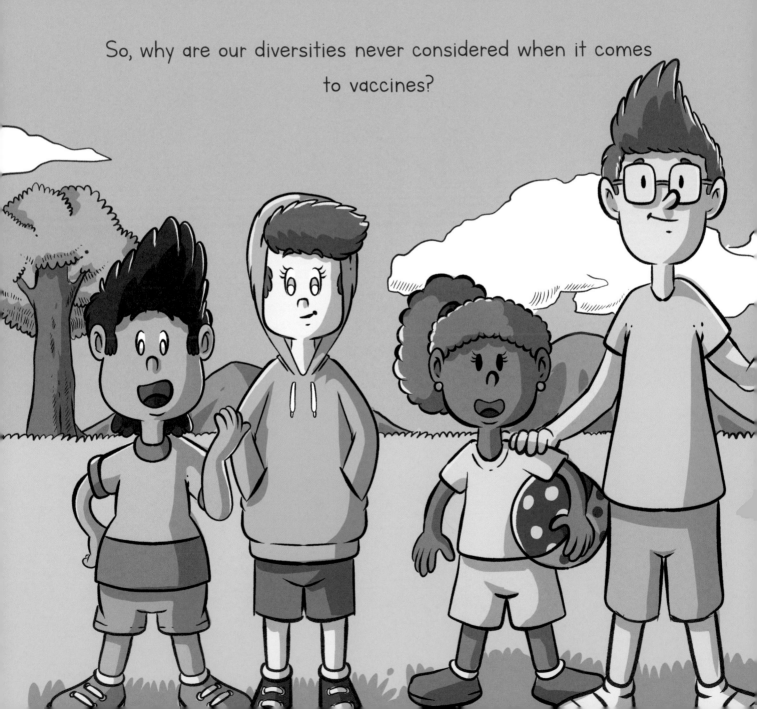

Even though everyone is unique in their own special way, we are each expected to get the same number of shots and the same exact dosage.

People are not 'one size fits all' when it comes to medication, so why is this approach used for vaccines?

It just doesn't make sense!

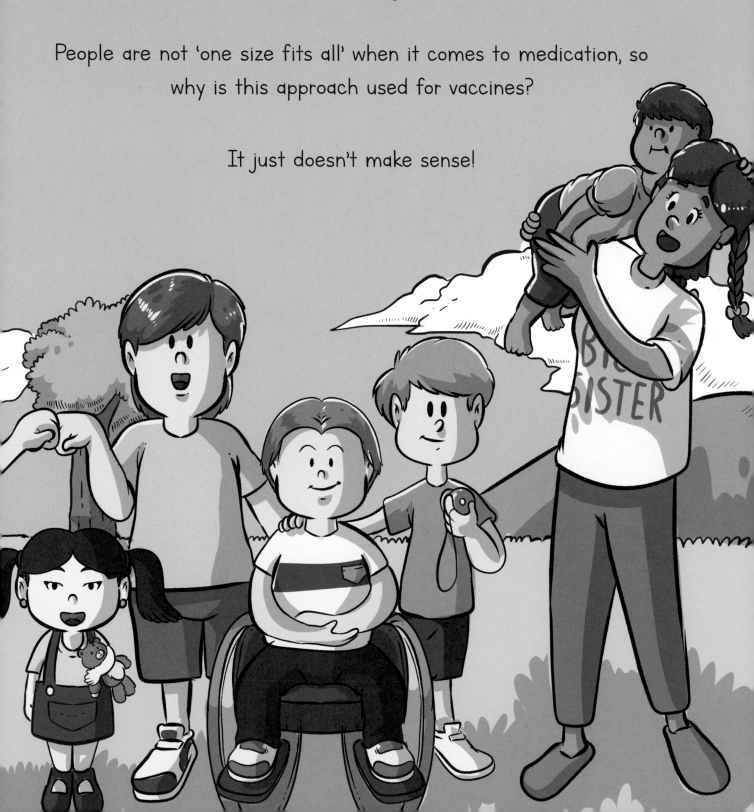

It is also interesting that vaccine trials have never compared the health of vaccinated kids to unvaccinated kids. This is called a placebo trial and is one of the most common ways that medical products are tested and proven safe. Yet, true placebo trials are rarely used to test vaccines.

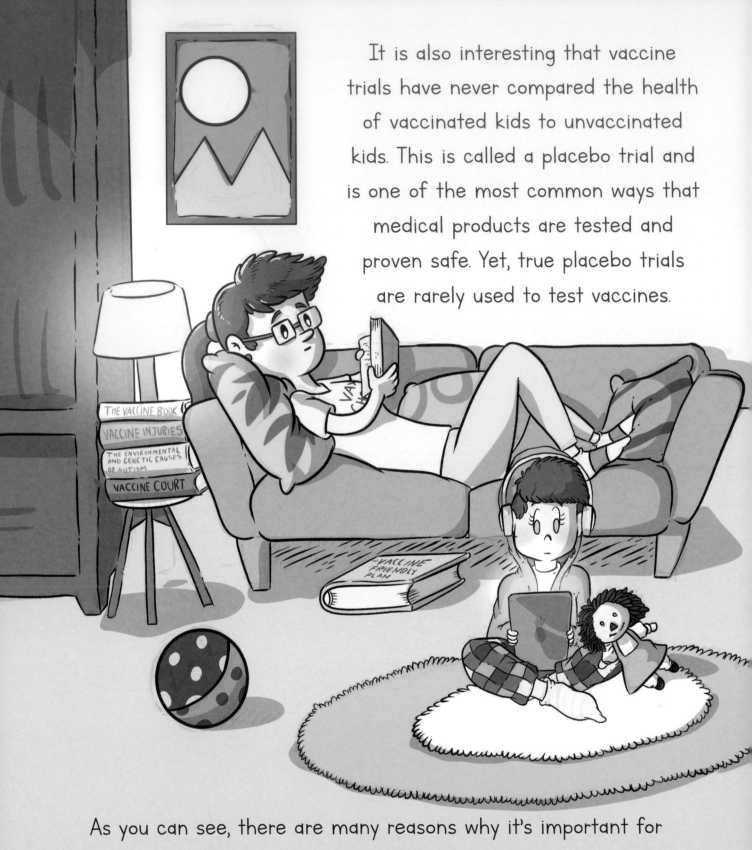

As you can see, there are many reasons why it's important for parents to research all they can when considering vaccinations for their children.

There are lots of great books, movies, and websites available with factual information about vaccine ingredients and possible side effects.

Some parents may even want to ask their doctor to discuss the vaccine insert paper that comes with each vaccine before choosing to vaccinate.

Doing all that research may sound like a lot of work, but I'm glad my parents took the time to do it for me.

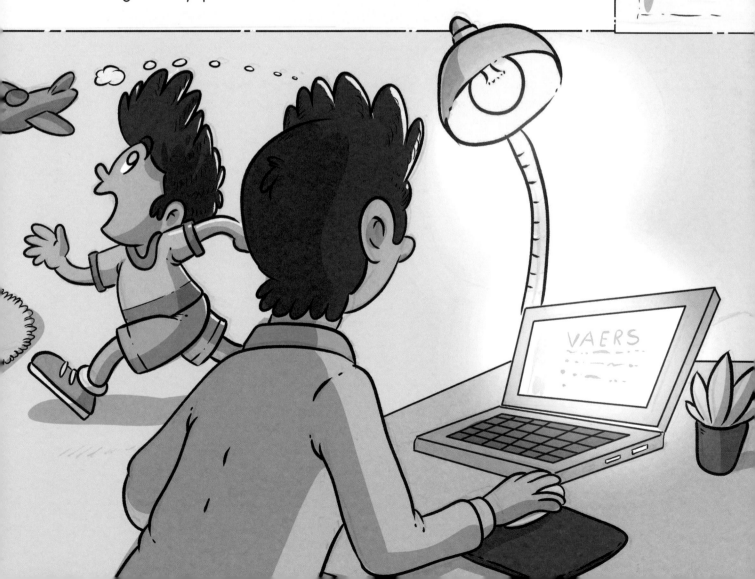

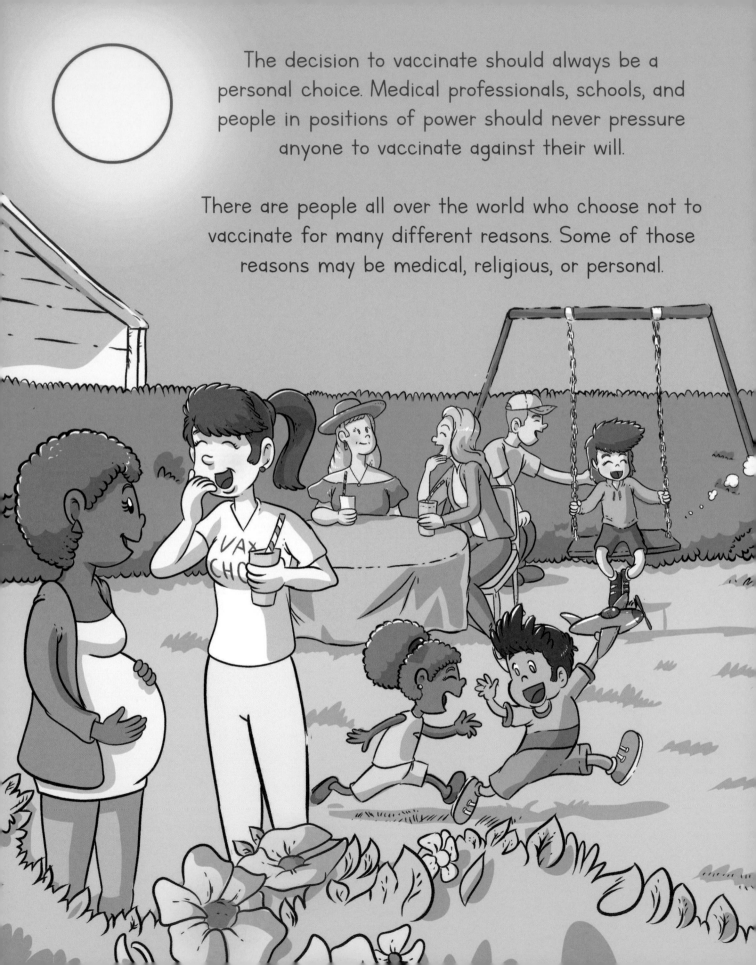

The decision to vaccinate should always be a personal choice. Medical professionals, schools, and people in positions of power should never pressure anyone to vaccinate against their will.

There are people all over the world who choose not to vaccinate for many different reasons. Some of those reasons may be medical, religious, or personal.

Whether someone chooses to get all the recommended vaccines, some vaccines, or none at all, the choice should always remain their own.

Some of my friends and family are vaccinated. Some of them are not. I love and respect them all equally, and they love me just as I am.

I'm unvaccinated and that's OK!

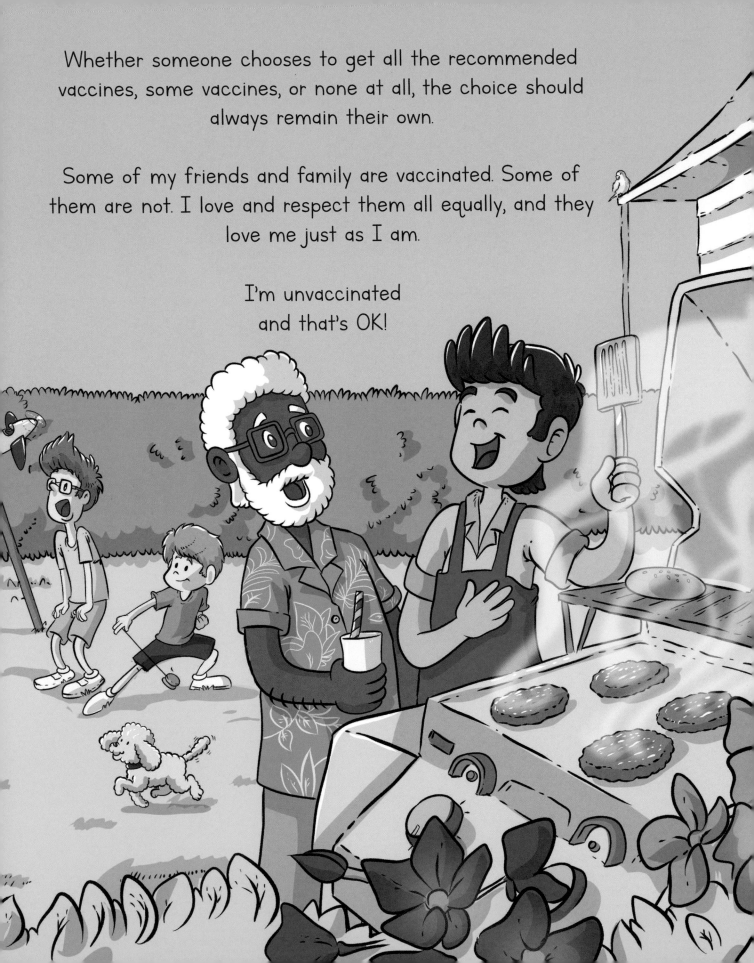

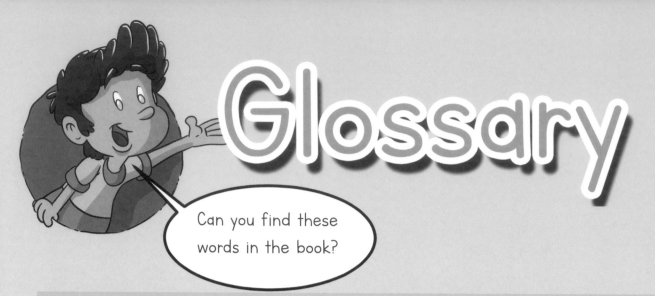

Glossary

Can you find these words in the book?

<u>Adverse reaction</u>: An adverse reaction, also referred to as an adverse event, is an undesirable side effect that may occur after vaccination. These reactions can range from mild, moderate, to severe. Adverse reactions may also be life-threatening and occasionally lead to death.

<u>Aluminum</u>: Aluminum salts, derived from aluminum, are adjuvants used in some vaccines. An adjuvant is a substance added to vaccines to help enhance the immune response, essentially turning your body's defenses on because it has detected a foreign or toxic substance.

<u>Antibiotics</u>: An antibiotic is a substance that stops the growth of bacteria. Antibiotics are used in vaccine production to help prevent bacterial contamination during manufacturing. As a result, small amounts of antibiotics may be present in some vaccines. Antibiotics used in vaccine production include neomycin, polymyxin B, streptomycin, and gentamicin.

<u>Autism</u>: Autism spectrum disorder (ASD) is a developmental condition that usually appears in early childhood and can last throughout one's life. It affects communication, social interaction, behavior, and self-regulation. "Spectrum" means that autism comes in different forms and levels of severity. Each person diagnosed with autism will have their own unique symptoms and challenges. The exact causes of autism are still being researched and are frequently debated. The National Institutes of Health (NIH) claims that if someone is susceptible to autism due to genetic mutations, then certain environmental situations, such as exposure to toxic chemicals, may cause autism in that person. Current data shows that one in thirty-six children has autism.

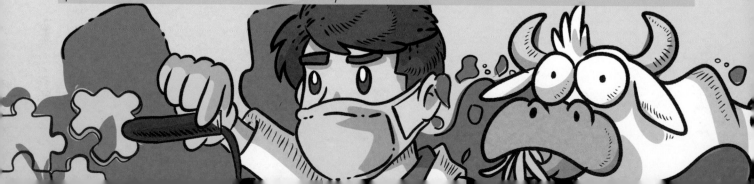

Cow serum: When viral vaccines are made, scientists often use cow serum, also referred to as "fetal bovine serum," as a protein source to grow the virus in. The Food and Drug Administration (FDA) claims that cows are used because they are large and commonly used for food. Animal-derived products for vaccine development may include amino acids, geletin, enzymes, and blood.

Encephalitis: Encephalitis is swelling, or inflammation, of the brain. It is commonly triggered after a person contracts certain viruses or bacteria. If the virus or bacteria ends up traveling to the spinal cord or brain, it causes inflammation. This inflammation produces the symptoms of encephalitis. In some cases, a person may experience encephalitis as a vaccine side effect.

Formaldehyde: Formaldehyde is a vaccine ingredient used to kill viruses or inactivate toxins during the manufacturing process. It is diluted during the vaccine manufacturing process; however, small amounts of formaldehyde may be found in some current vaccines. Formaldehyde is also commonly used in the manufacturing of resins, fertilizers, dyes, and embalming fluid. Excessive exposure to formaldehyde may cause cancer.

Homeschool: While most children attend traditional public or private school, a growing number of children are being homeschooled. Homeschooling is parent-directed education, in which parents educate their children at home with a customized educational curriculum to meet the child's needs. Today, there are a number of homeschool programs and resources that make homeschooling possible for every family, even those with full-time working parents.

Human cells: Scientists use specific cells to grow viruses to produce vaccines. Since viruses infect people, scientists discovered that they could use human cells to grow viruses for vaccine production. Some of these human cells come from fetal tissue. As a result, human diploid cells, including DNA and protein, may be present in some vaccines as a consequence of production methods.

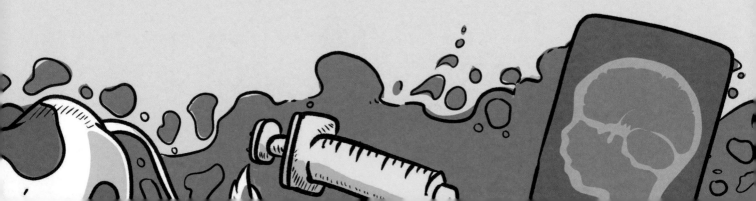

Immune system: Most people are born with a healthy immune system that helps to protect against diseases caused by pathogens such as viruses, bacteria, and parasites. The immune system is made up of specialized organs, cells, and tissues that work together to destroy foreign invaders. Some of the main organs involved in the immune system include the spleen, lymph nodes, thymus, and bone marrow.

Liability: Liability refers to the state of being responsible for something. In the 1980s, many vaccine manufacturers were being overwhelmed by vaccine injury lawsuits. As a result, many manufacturers stopped making vaccines. In fear of a vaccine shortage, Congress passed the National Childhood Vaccine Injury Act of 1986, protecting vaccine manufacturers from being liable of causing injury of death, thus allowing vaccines to continue being produced.

Monkey cells: Vaccine manufacturers specifically use Vero cells, which come from the kidneys of the African green monkey. These cells are used in the vaccine manufacturing process to grow specific viruses for viral vaccines.

Neurological issues: These are medical problems that may include the brain and spinal cord, as well as cranial and peripheral nerves, nerve roots, the autonomic nervous system, the neuromuscular junction, and muscles.

Organic: Organic refers to how certain foods are produced. Organic foods are grown or farmed without the use of artificial chemicals, such as human-made pesticides and fertilizers, and do not contain hormones, antibiotics, or genetically modified organisms (GMOs).

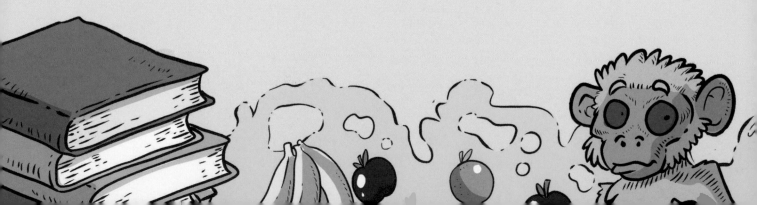

Pig gelatin: Also known as "porcine gelatin," this ingredient is used as a stabilizer to help vaccines remain stable and unaltered during transportation and storage. Gelatin used in vaccines is a protein which comes directly from the skin or connective tissue of pigs.

Placebo: A placebo is an inactive substance or treatment often used in clinical trials. A placebo-controlled trial compares a new treatment or medication with a placebo, which is usually in the form of a safe substance such as saline or a sugar pill.

Toxin: A toxin is a poisonous substance that may cause harm to your body.

Vaccine: A vaccine is a biological substance meant to cause the body's immune system to make antibodies to fight a particular pathogen. There are many different types of vaccines: inactivated, live-attenuated, messenger RNA (mRNA), subunit, recombinant, polysaccharide, conjugate, toxoid, and viral vector. Some vaccines contain weakened germs, a portion of a germ, inactivated or killed germs, a toxin made by the germ that causes a disease, or a molecule of messenger RNA, (mRNA), which uses the information in genes to instruct your body to make a protein of the germ.

Vaccine injury: Also called a vaccine-adverse event, a vaccine injury is caused by one or multiple vaccines. A vaccine injury may be caused by the vaccine itself or by medical error. Vaccine injuries can vary between mild and serious. Some vaccine injuries may even lead to death.

Vaccine insert: Sometimes referred to as a package insert, every vaccine comes with a tightly folded, multipage document with important information about the specific vaccine. This information often includes dosage, ingredients, possible side effects, results of clinical trials, specific warnings, possible allergic reactions, and much more. The purpose of the vaccine insert is to protect the pharmaceutical company from legal issues.

VAERS: Established in 1990, the Vaccine Adverse Event Reporting System (VAERS) is a passive, warning system used to detect vaccine-related risk factors, side effects, and track the occurrence of adverse events and vaccine-related deaths. VAERS is co-managed by the Centers for Disease Control and Prevention (CDC) and the US Food and Drug Administration (FDA). Healthcare professionals and vaccine manufacturers are required to report adverse events; yet many fail to do so.

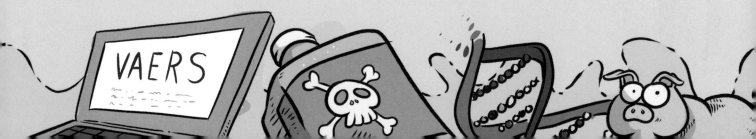

About the author

Dr. Shannon Kroner has a doctorate in Clinical Psychology and a master's in Special Education, with a focus in Educational Therapy. Her doctoral dissertation, entitled, *Childhood Vaccinations: The Development of an Educational Manual*, provides a psychological viewpoint of the ways in which parents make decisions regarding vaccinations for their children.

When Dr. Kroner first began working with special needs families in 2001 as a Floortime therapist and behaviorist, she discovered many parents sharing similar stories about their children's disabilities having occurred shortly after receiving a vaccine. Then, in 2009, while pregnant, Dr. Kroner personally suffered a vaccine injury after receiving a preservative-free flu shot. Believing it was safer than others because it was preservative-free, she got the vaccine, but suffered a serious reaction that landed her in the emergency room. Upon hearing so many personal vaccine injury stories and then experiencing her own adverse reaction, Dr. Kroner decided it was time to seriously research vaccines and encourage others to do the same.

In 2019, following vaccine mandate laws that removed both religious and medical exemptions in California, Dr. Kroner founded the organization, Freedom of Religion - United Solutions (FOR-US). Serving as its Executive Director, she has united faith leaders of many faiths to protect the religious freedom of vaccine choice and has helped thousands of individuals obtain religious vaccine exemptions.

As a public speaker, advocate, author, wife, and mother, Dr. Kroner understands the importance of protecting vaccine choice and educating today's children as they pave the way towards a brighter tomorrow.

For more information on Dr. Kroner, please visit her website www.drshannonkroner.com.

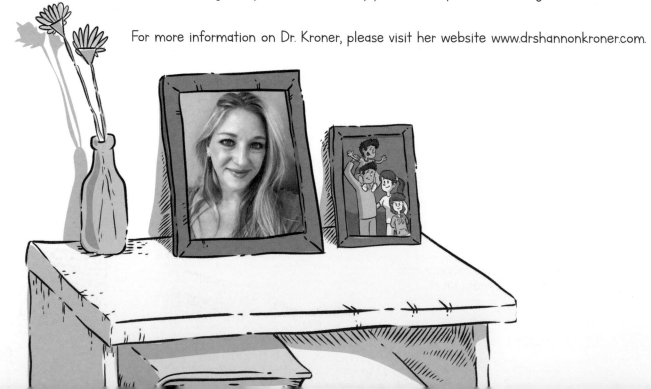

SUGGESTED RESOURCES

RESOURCE RECOMMENDATIONS

CDC Pink Book: Epidemiology of Vaccine Preventable Diseases
www.cdc.gov/vaccines/pubs/pinkbook/chapters.html

Childhood Vaccine Schedule
"Immunization Schedules for 18 and Younger." Centers for Disease Control and Prevention, 10 Feb. http://www.cdc.gov/vaccines/schedules/hcp/imz/child-adolescent.html

Vaccine Ingredients
Institute for Vaccine Safety || Components: Excipients. hopkinsvaccine.org/components-Excipients.htm.

National Vaccine Injury Compensation Program
About the National Vaccine Injury Compensation Program | HRSA. 1 Mar. 2023, www.hrsa.gov/vaccine-compensation

Reporting a vaccine injury to the Vaccine Adverse Event Reporting System (VAERS)
Vaccine Adverse Event Reporting System (VAERS). vaers.hhs.gov

Kern, J. K., Geier, D. A., Sykes, L. K., & Geier, M. R. (2016). *Relevance of Neuroinflammation and Encephalitis in Autism.* Frontiers in cellular neuroscience, 9, 519

BOOK RECOMMENDATIONS

Dissolving Illusions: Disease, Vaccines and the Forgotten History by Suzanne Humpharies and Roman Bystrianyk (2013)

The Environmental and Genetic Causes of Autism by James Lyons-Weiler (2016)

The Vaccine Book: Making the Right Decision for Your Child by Robert W. Sears (2011)

The Vaccine Court 2.0: Revised and Updated: The Dark Truth of America's Vaccine Injury Compensation Program by Wayne Rohde (2021)

Vaccine Epidemic: How Corporate Greed, Biased Science, and Coercive Government Threaten Our Human Rights, Our Health, and Our Children by Louise Kuo Habakus (2011)

Vaccine Injuries: Documented Adverse Reactions to Vaccines by Lou Conte and Tony Lyons (2014)

Vaccine-Friendly Plan: Dr. Paul's Safe and Effective Approach to Immunity and Health-from Pregnancy Through Your Child's Teen Years by Paul Thomas and Jennifer Margulis (2016)

Vaccines, Autoimmunity, and the Changing Nature of Childhood Illness by Thomas Cowan (2018)

Vax-Unvax: Let the Science Speak by Brian Hooker and Robert F. Kennedy Jr. (2023)

WEBSITE RECOMMENDATIONS

Know your rights: https://icandecide.org/

Vaccine exemptions: https://forunitedsolutions.org/

Latest news: https://thehighwire.com/

Research studies: https://ipaknowledge.org/

Educational rights: https://www.perk-group.com/

Find a doctor: https://physiciansforinformedconsent.org/

Homeschool info: https://www.samsorbo.com/

Podcast: https://drtenpenny.com/

Vaccine info: https://www.stopmandatoryvaccination.com/

Vaccine info: https://childrenshealthdefense.org/

The Spellers Method: https://spellers.com/

Report a vaccine injury: https://vaers.hhs.gov/esub/index.jsp

MOVIE RECOMMENDATIONS

Bought
Sacrificial Virgins
SPELLERS
The Silent Epidemic: The Untold Story of Vaccines
VAXXED: From Cover Up to Catastrophe
VAXXED II: The People's Truth

For more resource recommendations scan the QR code or visit
www.drshannonkroner.com

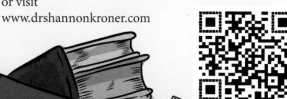

Visit our website at www.skyhorsepublishing.com.
10 9 8 7 6 5 4 3

Manufactured in the United States of America, May 2023
This product conforms to CPSIA 2008

Library of Congress Cataloging-in-Publication Data is available on file.

Hardcover ISBN: 978-1-5107-7819-1
Ebook ISBN: 978-1-5107-7820-7

Cover design by Manfred Calderón
Cover illustration by Manfred Calderón

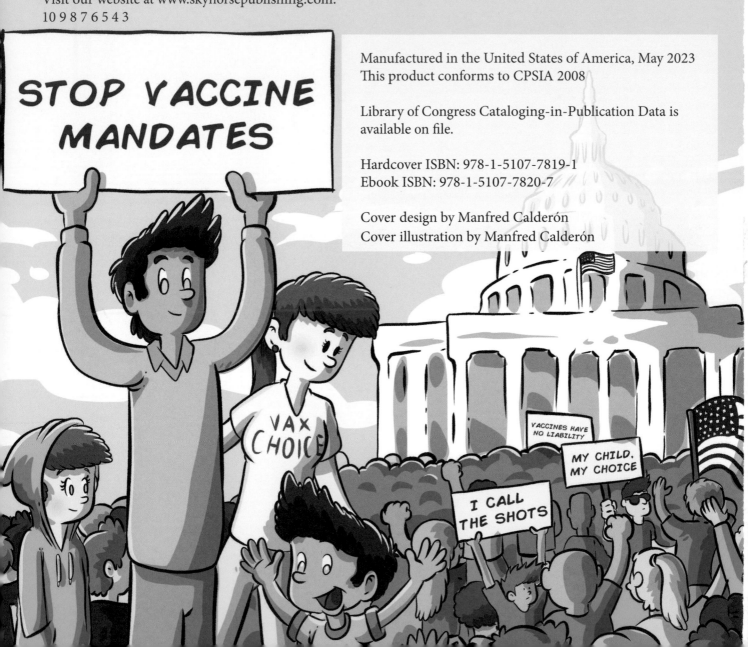